The 28 Da

ENERGIZE

Christine Green

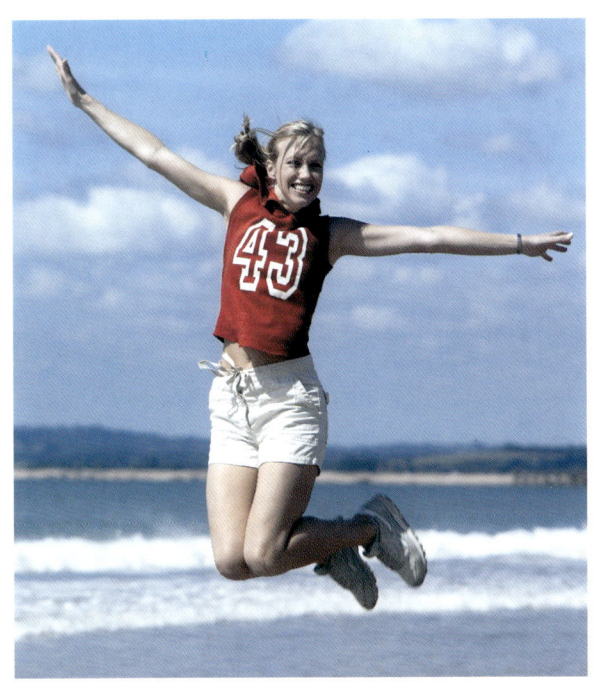

p

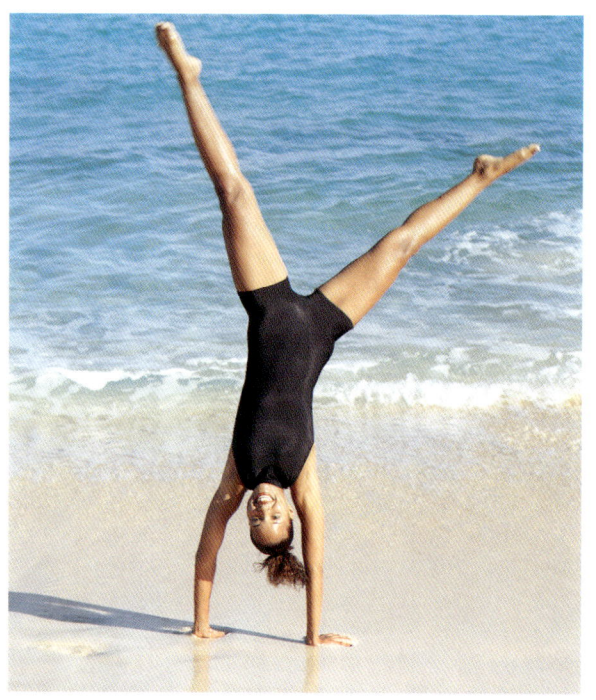

This is a Parragon Publishing Book

First published by Parragon 2002

Parragon Publishing
Queen Street House
4 Queen Street
Bath BA1 1HE, UK

Copyright © Parragon 2002

Designed, produced and packaged by
Stonecastle Graphics Limited

Text by Christine Green
Edited by Gillian Haslam
Designed by Sue Pressley and Paul Turner
Commissioned photography by Roddy Paine

ISBN 0-75256-798-5

Printed in China

Disclaimer

The exercises and advice detailed in this book
assume that you are a normally healthy adult.
Therefore the author, publishers, their servants, or
agents cannot accept responsibility for loss or
damage suffered by individuals as a result of
following advice or attempting an exercise or
treatment referred to in this book. It is strongly
recommended that individuals intending to
undertake an exercise program and any change of
diet do so following consultation with their medical
practitioner.

Contents

What Do We Mean By "Energize?"

Does this sound familiar? Do you normally wake up in the mornings feeling just as tired as when you went to bed? Do you skip breakfast and then by mid-morning find yourself reaching for the cookies?

Is lunch normally a quick sandwich and cup of coffee, only for you to find that by mid-afternoon your energy levels are dipping and so you need another cookie and another cup of coffee? This describes a common but far from healthy lifestyle that could be draining your energy resources and preventing your body from working at its optimum.

If this reflects your life, this 28-day energize program is just what you need. By the end of the four weeks you will look healthier, feel healthier and your batteries will be fully recharged.

What causes lack of energy?

There are many contributory factors that can lead to a feeling of lassitude and lack of energy. If you constantly feel tired and have checked with your doctor that there are no underlying medical conditions, perhaps it is time to consider other possible factors.

Bad diet

Fad dieting, erratic eating patterns, skipping meals or simply choosing a bad diet can play havoc with your overall well-being, draining your energy resources and leaving you feeling totally exhausted.

Persuade yourself never to skip a meal, especially breakfast first thing in the morning when the body is

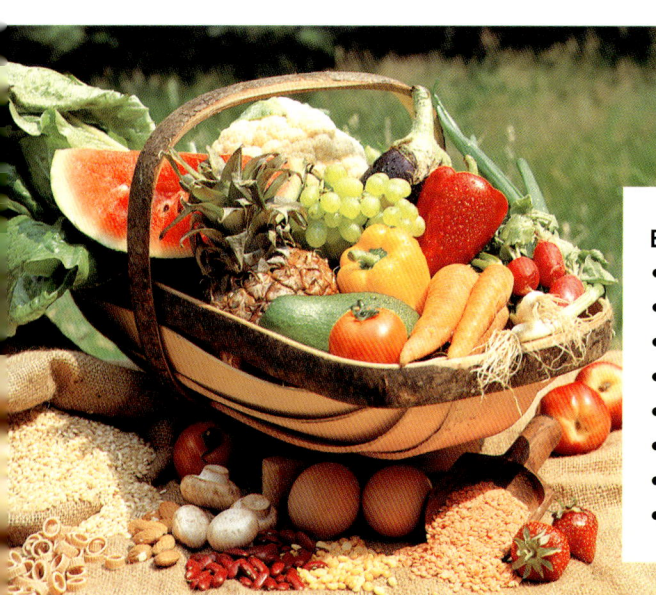

Each day throughout your 28-day program you should:
- Always eat breakfast
- Take one dose of aloe vera with your breakfast drink
- Eat three meals a day
- Take a multivitamin supplement for the first 15 days
- Drink at least 3 pints of water
- Eat at least three portions of fresh fruit
- Eat at least three portions of vegetables
- Eat one portion of a non-dairy product

at its lowest ebb and needs fuelling after a period of rest. Skipping meals during the day, surviving on cups of coffee and then eating a large meal in the evening, is very bad for you. Depriving the body of food during the day will deplete blood sugar levels and leave you feeling tired and even slightly light-headed. Your aim must be to eat three meals a day combined with low-fat healthy snacks in between if you feel peckish.

Stress

Whether it is caused by your job or the daily commitments of a busy housewife and mother, stress is an unavoidable fact of modern living. We all need a certain amount of stress in our lives in order to motivate us to do things, to get up in the morning or to pay the bills on time, but problems occur when stress works its way into the very fabric of your life and you end up with chronic physical and often emotional problems, including:

- Anxiety
- Depression
- Digestive problems
- Headaches
- Insomnia
- Irritable bowel syndrome
- Lack of energy

Stress isn't normally life-threatening but that doesn't mean that you should allow it to dominate your life. Learning to recognize and deal with stress is an invaluable lesson that you must learn. Coping with stress often involves doing something to take your mind off the immediate problem or situation – go out for a walk, listen to some music, do some housework, try anything that will distract your mind and help you to relax.

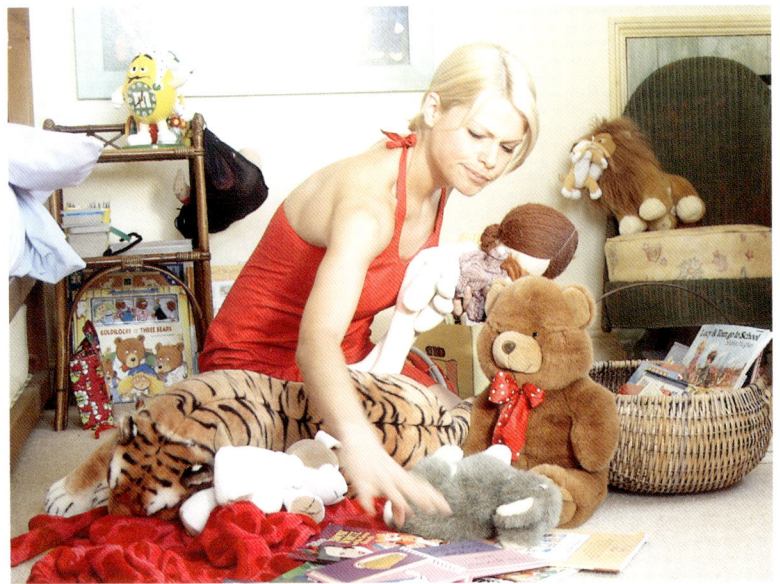

Whenever the body is experiencing stress, energy levels are sapped and several important nutrients, namely vitamins B and C and zinc, are used up. The only way to replenish that store is by eating foods containing high levels of these essential nutrients.

Vitamin B helps to maintain a healthy nervous system and release energy. It is found in potatoes, green vegetables, tomatoes, fresh and dried fruit, wheatgerm, wholegrain cereals, brown rice, eggs, dairy products, seafood, lean meat, liver, kidney, poultry, peas, beans, lentils, nuts, and seeds.

Vitamin C helps the body to protect itself against possible infection. It is found in fresh fruits (particularly citrus fruit, i.e. oranges, grapefruit etc.), blackcurrants, fruit juices, and fresh vegetables.

Zinc helps the body to resist possible infection. It is found in liver, red meat, egg yolks, dairy produce, wholegrain cereals, oysters, and other shellfish.

Complex carbohydrates help to increase energy levels and relax the mind. They are found in bread, rice, pulses, oats, pasta, and potatoes.

Alcohol

Most people enjoy the odd glass of wine or beer, but when alcohol becomes a prop to cope with an underlying problem, it takes on a very different aspect. Not only does alcohol act as a sedative, it also dehydrates you. That glass of wine drunk at lunchtime may well cause you to feel tired by mid-afternoon and one too many drinks taken at night may well cause restless sleep resulting in low energy levels the following morning.

The message is quite simple – take everything in moderation. One or two glasses of wine with a meal is fine; if you are going out for a couple of drinks in the evening, then make sure that you drink plenty of water before going to bed to prevent possible dehydration.

Sleep

We go to sleep in order to rest both the mind and body and to awaken fresh and invigorated the following morning. However, for some people bedtime is a nightmare because they spend most of the night

Alcohol

The recommended weekly limit of 21 units of alcohol for men and 14 units for women, who are not pregnant, should ideally be spread over the full course of the week.

1 unit = $\frac{1}{2}$ pint of beer = a small glass of wine = a small glass of sherry = a small glass of spirits

lying awake staring into space. Sleeplessness or insomnia is a condition for which there are numerous treatments readily available, but before going to the doctor or pharmacy, why not try some self-help methods:

✓ Take some exercise during the day to keep the body active and to prepare it for rest at bedtime

✓ Try some relaxation methods to help you unwind

✓ Avoid drinking any stimulants, such as coffee or tea, preferably from early evening onwards

✓ Eat a healthy, balanced diet to encourage the body to function more effectively

✓ Take a good book to bed with you

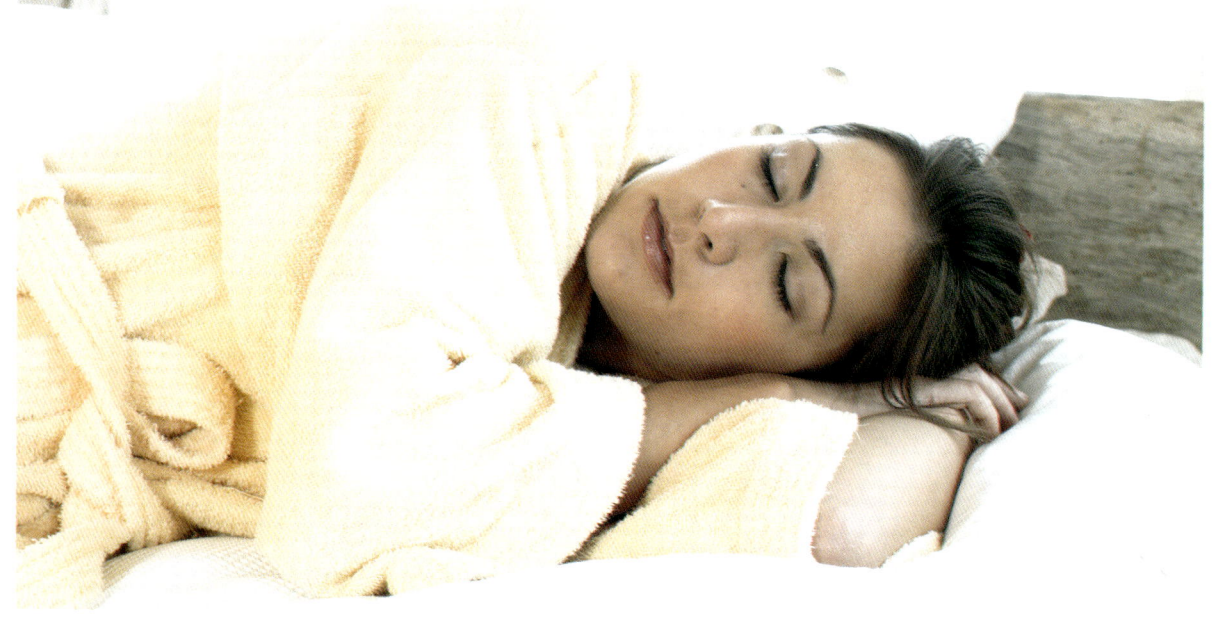

Smoking

To maintain a high level of energy, the body requires a good supply of oxygen. Smoking reduces the amount of oxygen the body absorbs. Imagine every time you reach for a cigarette to give you an instant "high," you are in fact doing the opposite. So give up smoking!

Signs of lack of energy:
- Inability to sleep
- Indigestion
- Irritability
- Lack of concentration
- Low blood sugar
- Mood swings
- Tiredness

Following the 28-day energize program

The endless cycle of tiredness and feeling below par can become a daily way of life. But it needn't be that way. It is possible to free yourself from this routine and:

✓ Break the cycle of tiredness
✓ Enhance your brain power
✓ Help maintain stamina levels throughout the day
✓ Help you to find your natural, healthy body weight
✓ Leave you feeling invigorated and rejuvenated
✓ And put a spring back in your step!

Surprise friends, family, workmates (and more importantly yourself) by showing everyone how energetic and healthy you feel after following this 28-day program.

To succeed on the program:
- Adopt a positive attitude from the beginning
- Stay focused throughout
- Regard each new day as a new challenge
- Keep it exciting by adding different treatments from time to time
- Experiment with different foods
- And don't forget, pamper yourself

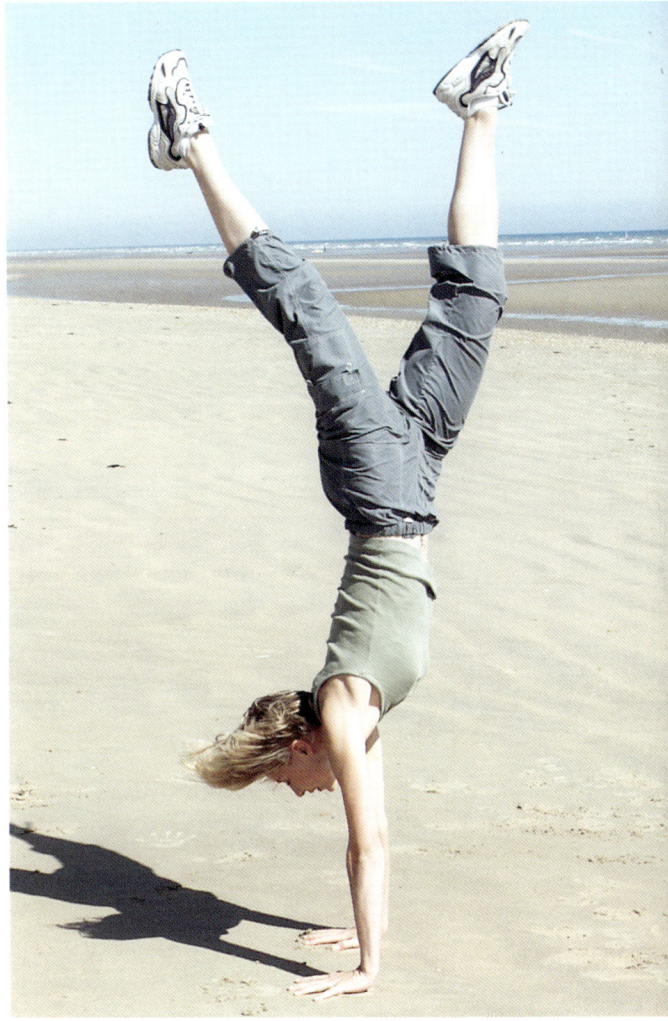

You are not advised to go on the energy program if:
- You are pregnant or breastfeeding
- You are seeing your doctor for some medical condition
- You have anaemia
- You have Type 1 diabetes
- You are underweight
- You are experiencing extreme stress
- You are taking prescription medicines that cannot be discontinued

Food For Energy

An important lesson that you will learn while on this 28-day program is how to recognize foods that are good for you and those that are not, those that improve your performance and those that impair it.

Once you can easily distinguish between the good foods from the bad foods, you will be able to eliminate the "bad guys" from your diet and replace them with "good guys."

Energy is the driving force the body needs to:
✓ Enable muscles to move and carry out physical activities
✓ Maintain our normal body temperature
✓ Carry out essential physical functions, such as breathing, heartbeat and metabolism
✓ Promote tissue growth and repair

The body derives this energy from its intake of food. The main energy-producing nutrients are contained in three different food groups – carbohydrates, proteins, and fats.

Carbohydrates
The main function of carbohydrates is to provide energy for the body. During digestion, carbohydrates are converted into glucose which is then absorbed into the bloodstream. The body uses the glucose for energy. If energy is not required immediately, it is stored in the muscles and the liver as glycogen where it remains available to be converted into glucose when extra energy is required.

Carbohydrate-rich foods:
- Baked beans
- Barley
- Brown rice
- Cereal
- Couscous
- Fresh fruit
- Grains
- Honey
- Juices
- Muesli
- Oat crackers
- Pasta
- Pitta bread
- Porridge oats
- Potatoes
- Pulses
- Rice cakes
- Rice flour
- Rye bread
- Sweetcorn
- Tortillas
- Vegetables
- Wholemeal bread/rolls
- Wholemeal flour

Proteins
They are invaluable to the body principally for the role they play in repair and maintenance of the tissues, muscles and blood cells. An excess intake of protein is either converted into energy or converted into fat and stored in the body for emergency use.

Protein-rich foods:
- Brown bread
- Butter
- Chicken
- Chickpeas, lentils
- Cooking oils
- Dairy products, i.e. milk, cheese, yogurt, goat's milk cheese
- Fish – fresh, frozen, canned
- Kidney
- Liver
- Meat – bacon, beef, lamb, pork
- Meat products – beefburgers, sausages
- Nuts
- Quorn – meat substitute
- Soya
- Turkey

Fats

The role fats play in the body's energy budget is to supply it with a concentrated source of energy and also fatty acids vital for the maintenance of a healthy skin and the regulation of body functions.

Fat-rich foods: these should be eaten sparingly

- Cakes
- Desserts
- Ice cream
- Chips
- Sweeteners

If you have a sweet tooth, then avoid sugar and artificial sweeteners, instead try healthier alternatives:

- Blackstrap molasses
- Honey
- Fructose powder (fruit sugar)
- Real maple syrup

Foods that are good and bad for maintaining energy levels

Bad guys:	Good guys:
Sugary cereals	Porridge, muesli
Pasties, pies, sausages	Fish, poultry, lamb
Cookies, chocolate	Bananas, dried fruit
French fries	Baked potatoes
Salted nuts, crisps	Sesame seeds, fresh nuts
White bread	Wholemeal, brown bread
Sweet fizzy drinks	Fresh juice, water
Cooking oil	Extra virgin olive oil
Margarine	Butter/non-hydrogenated margarine
Packaged orange juice	Home-made apple/grape juice
Coffee, tea	Water, freshly squeezed fruit or vegetable juice, herbal tea
Dairy milk	Soya milk
Cow's milk cheese	Sheep's or goat's milk cheese
Beef or pork	Lean lamb, lamb's liver

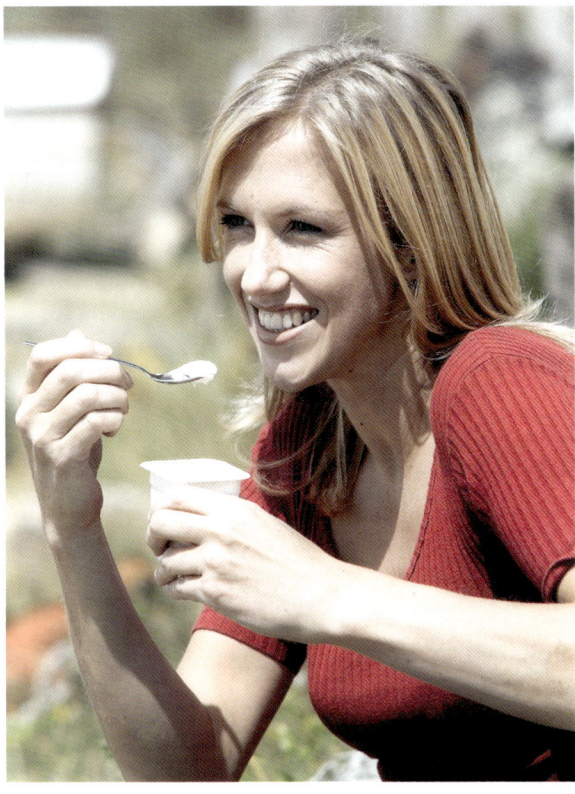

Maintaining energy levels

Most people enjoy the instant buzz you get after eating a bar of chocolate or drinking a cup of coffee. You instantly feel re-energized both physically and mentally. Yet those feelings are short-lived because once the initial "lift" has waned, energy levels plummet.

However, on the other side of the equation from those foods that can drain energy levels, there are other foods that can keep energy levels evenly balanced. Here is a list showing you some examples of the "bad guys" – those foods that give you an instant, but short-lived, energy boost – while on the opposite side are the "good guys", the healthier energy-boosting alternatives.

Write them out on a piece of paper and stick it up on your kitchen wall, so that you can refer to the list throughout your program.

Eating for energy

While on the 28-day program your main aim is to eat for energy so:

• Always eat breakfast

• Reduce, or better still cut out, stimulants such as coffee, chocolate or sugar

• Do not go for long periods through the day without eating something

• Eating small meals little and often puts less strain on the digestive system and burns calories far more efficiently

• If you find that your energy levels are low, increase the protein content of your diet. Often protein foods will satisfy the appetite for longer than carbohydrates

What to buy

Shopping for food can be a nightmare, especially if you are trying to keep a mental note of those foods that will provide extra energy and those that are depriving your body of energy, however tempting they may look.

Here are some guidelines to make that choice a little easier.

Fresh fruit

Fruit provides most of our daily intake of vitamin C. Aim to eat two or three pieces of fresh fruit each day.

• Apples
• Apricots
• Bananas
• Blackberries
• Blackcurrants
• Blueberries
• Cherries
• Dried figs
• Golden raisins

• Grapefruit
• Grapes
• Figs
• Kiwi fruit
• Lemons
• Limes
• Mangos
• Melons
• Nectarines

• Papaya
• Passionfruit
• Peaches
• Pears
• Pineapple
• Raspberries
• Strawberries

Vegetables

Vegetables are good foods. They are packed with essential fiber, vitamins and minerals. Aim to include at least two or three portions each day.

• Artichokes
• Asparagus
• Avocados
• Bamboo shoots
• Beansprouts
• Beet
• Broccoli
• Brussels sprouts
• Cabbage (dark green is healthier)
• Calabrese
• Capsicums

• Carrots
• Cauliflower
• Celeriac
• Chicory
• Chives
• Eggplant
• Endive
• Garlic
• Kale
• Leeks
• Lettuce (dark green is healthier)
• Mange-tout

• Mushrooms
• Mustard and cress
• Onions (scallions too)
• Shallots
• Spinach
• Squash
• Swedes
• Tomatoes
• Turnips
• Watercress
• Zucchini

The "try to avoid at all times" foods

If at all possible, avoid the following foods which may give you an instant high, but then several hours later you will feel the lows.

• Beef (unless organic)
• Chocolate
• Cheese – colored, smoked, processed
• Cow's milk – drink sparingly
• Diet drinks
• Diet foods
• Fizzy drinks
• Hydrogenated oils
• Ice-cream

• Low-fat foods with lots of additives
• Margarine spreads
• Peanuts
• Pork (unless organic)
• Refined white flour
• Salty foods
• Sugar
• Sugar-coated cereals
• Wheat-based breakfast foods

Supplements

This 28-day energize program is not a diet; there is no calorie counting involved, just sensible healthy eating combined with a disciplined exercise program. At the beginning of the program you may well benefit from including a daily multivitamin supplement.

Experts are convinced that supplements are invaluable for providing the essential support our bodies need to cope with the energy-draining effects of modern day life.

Certain vitamins and minerals are essential for helping the body to produce energy. Many of them can be found in the "good guys" food list.

Aloe vera

A daily dose of aloe vera is used as a digestive tonic and is reputed to raise energy levels and enhance well-being. Take it daily mixed with fruit juice as a pre-breakfast drink.

Fast foods

Convenient and quick, the perfect standby, we seem to have become a generation of convenience food eaters, whether it is a beefburger dripping with tomato catsup, a plate of chips in salt, or a frozen ready-made meal packed with lots of additives and preservatives.

The occasional takeaway or frozen meal is fine, but a diet based mainly on such foods is badly deficient in a number of essential nutrients. The dishes are also high in calories, sodium, and fat.

If you really can't cope without a burger, then limit yourself to one as a special treat at the weekend and even then try to choose healthier options:

✓ Ask for small plain burgers, instead of big ones
✓ Miss out on the melted cheese, mayonnaise and other selected toppings
✓ Have a plain glass of milk instead of a milkshake
✓ Instead of fries, order a side salad

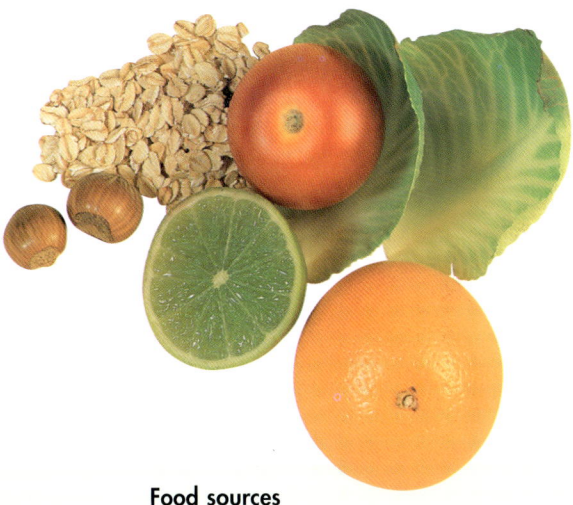

Nutrient	Role	Food sources
Iron	Needed for manufacturing red blood cells	Red meat, sardines, egg yolk, leafy vegetables
Zinc	Essential for maintaining a healthy immune system	Grains, nuts, fish, red meat, peanuts
Magnesium	Essential for building healthy bones	Green vegetables, wholegrain cereals, nuts
B vitamins	Essential for releasing energy from food	Broccoli, nuts, yeast, wholemeal bread
Vitamin C	Essential for healthy gums, teeth, skin, bones etc	Oranges, kiwi fruit, tomatoes
Vitamin E	Weakens unstable substances that can cause damage to cells	Green vegetables, nuts, vegetable oils

Drinking For Energy

Do you recognize this scenario? Get up in the morning, grab a cup of coffee before dashing off to work or getting the children ready for school. Mid-morning, feeling tired, time for another cup or two of coffee. Lunchtime, no time for lunch so grab another cup of coffee and a chocolate cookie...

If you can identify with this pattern of behavior, then you are by no means alone. Probably 80 per cent of the population crawl out of bed in the morning, gulp down a cup of coffee before dashing off to work or getting the children off to school, only to find that by mid-morning they are "dead on their feet" and in desperate need of something to keep them going. One cup of coffee can seem the perfect pick-me-up, but if you drink more than six cups a day, you are spiralling into caffeine dependency, so perhaps it is time to consider gradually weaning yourself off the stuff and replacing it with herbal tea.

What to drink

Maintaining a healthy balance of fluid in the body is important, provided that it is the right type of fluid. Experts recommend that we should aim to drink at least 3 pints of water a day to help clean out toxins and keep our bodies in tip-top condition.

A glass of hot water with a squeeze of lemon or lime added to it taken first thing in the morning is ideal for refreshing the mouth and kick-starting the body into action. But some people tend to prefer a glass of a sweet fizzy drink, or a cup of black coffee – neither of which is healthy and neither of which will sustain energy levels.

Although we say that everything can be taken in moderation while on the 28-day energize program,

there are some drinks that should definitely be avoided or at least limited.

Good	Bad
Fresh juice	Alcohol
Fresh vegetable juice	Coffee
Herbal tea	Sweet fizzy drinks
Low-calorie drinks	
Milk	
Water	

Fact A 11$\frac{1}{2}$ fl oz can of non-diet cola drink contains over seven teaspoons of sugar!

Fact The caffeine in coffee stimulates the brain and keeps you awake, but a high regular intake, i.e. more than eight cups a day, may well increase the risk of osteoporosis in later life. It causes migraine in those susceptible to it and can also be addictive.

Fact Drinking excessive amounts of alcohol destroys important vitamins A, C, and E that are needed for general health and also stamina.

Sports drinks

It may be tempting to buy commercial "isotonic" sports drinks that contain levels of salts and sugars for energy. A less expensive, and just as effective, alternative is to dilute fruit juice 1:1 with water.

Making your own energy drinks

Fresh is best, even when it comes to drinks, so why spend money on buying expensive pre-packaged "fresh juice" when you can make it at home for less than half the cost and with the added knowledge that you know that what the drink contains is only the best!

Both fresh fruit and vegetables are bursting with so much natural goodness that the benefits of consuming them are fundamental to good health. Once you begin drinking them, you will physically feel much healthier, your skin will become clearer, your eyes will sparkle and your hair shine. After all, what better way is there of ensuring that the body gets all the vitamins, minerals, and enzymes it needs in a form that is readily absorbed into the body? And so even if you don't fancy eating any fruit or vegetables on some days, you can still make sure you have your daily quota by drinking it out of a glass.

Anytime of the day drinks

Appetizing apple Chop up two medium-sized apples and pop them into a juicer. There is no need to remove the core or seeds.

Strawberry juice Take a punnet of strawberries, wash and then pluck off the green stalks before putting the strawberries into the juicer whole. Blend them to make a delicious summer drink.

Energy cocktail

1 banana
1 mango
1 teaspoon honey
Half a medium-sized pineapple

Make your own special cocktail for when your energy levels are flagging – simply pop all the ingredients into a blender and whiz them together. Within minutes you will have a deliciously tasty drink.

Red as a beet

If you fancy your quota of vegetables in a glass, then beet, which is packed with vitamins and minerals, makes a strong and tasty drink, especially when cucumber is added.

4oz raw beetroot
10oz cucumber or half a large one

Wash any soil from the beet. Remove any hairy roots, then slice and pop the pieces into the juicer. Do not peel the cucumber, simply rinse the skin in water. Slice it into pieces and place it together with the beet in the juicer.

Pep up

4 oranges
1 lemon
1 teaspoon honey
Ice cubes

Mix the juice of the oranges and lemon into a tumbler, adding one teaspoon of honey. Serve with ice for a wonderfully energizing and refreshing drink packed with vitamin C.

Banana whiz

2 bananas, chopped
4 oranges
1 pot of low-fat natural yogurt

Into a blender add the two chopped bananas, the flesh of four oranges and the pot of yogurt. Blend until it turns into a purée and then serve.

Energy Recipes

The great thing about the Energize program is that you can eat a wide variety of healthy

foods that will make you feel good and maintain your energy levels throughout the day.

You will be amazed at the difference changing your daily diet will make

to your overall sense of well-being.

Remember, you don't have to eat huge meals – small frequent snacks throughout the day are often better in helping to maintain a constant energy supply and to avoid fatigue setting in. Nutritionists recommend that you aim to consume 50 per cent of your daily calories in the form of carbohydrates, 10-15 per cent in the form of proteins, and 35 per cent in the form of fats.

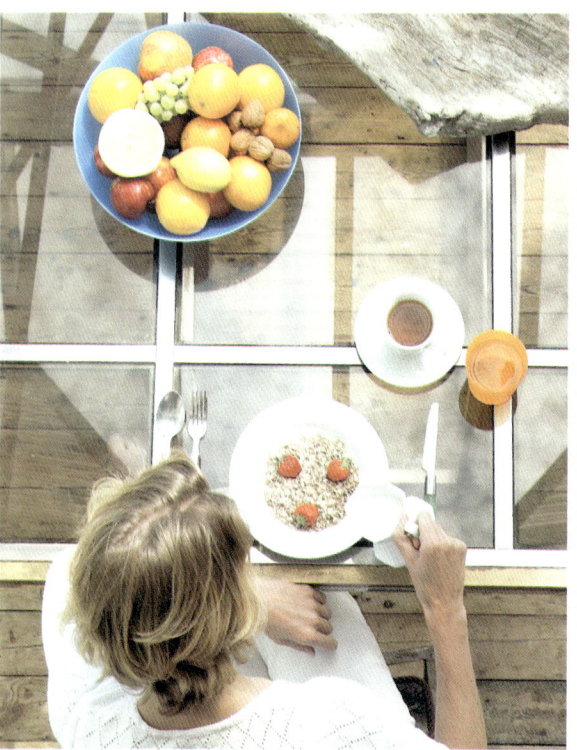

Breakfast recipes

The longest gap between any of the daily meals is the period between dinner and breakfast the following morning. During the eight or so hours that you are sleeping, the body is still actively working, repairing cells, and keeping the heart and organs functioning, and it derives energy from the store of sugar or glucose held in the blood, liver, and muscles. It is small wonder that by sunrise, and with more than half of the body's glucose used up, it needs refuelling. This emphasizes the importance of a good breakfast.

If you skip breakfast just to enjoy another 20 minutes' lie-in, the chances are that you will function perfectly well for the first few hours of the day, but once your blood sugar levels drop, poor concentration, lethargy and irritability will set in and by mid-morning you will probably be eating your third chocolate cookie or drinking your fifth cup of coffee.

From now on, things are going to change! Make a determined effort every day to have a good breakfast; prepare it the night before if that's easier.

Breakfast choices Stay clear of foods that are high in sugar, such as doughnuts or sugary cereals. Although they provide a quick energy buzz, this will leave you feeling tired a few hours later.

The ideal breakfast foods contain a combination of carbohydrate, fiber, and protein, each helping to stabilize blood sugar levels. Try these suggestions:

• Chopped apple with unsweetened yogurt and ground sesame seeds sprinkled over the top

• Scrambled eggs with rye toast

• Mix a chopped banana and a small pot of low-fat yogurt with some unsweetened muesli

• Yogurt with wheatgerm, honey, and stewed dried apricots on top

• Toasted bagel with cottage cheese

• A muffin topped with a little fat-free cheese and broiled until brown. Serve with a glass of freshly squeezed orange juice

• A generous serving of high-fiber cereal. Topped with fruit, such as golden raisins or raspberries, with 1 per cent milk for a perfect, nutritious, quick breakfast.

Never skip breakfast

• It is the most important meal of the day and helps to refuel the body after it has rested

• It will discourage you from grabbing a sugary snack mid-morning

• It will help to maintain your sugar levels

• Research studies have found that adults who eat a balanced breakfast sustain better mental performance throughout the day

Liquid breakfast

Many people baulk at the idea of eating any solid food in the morning, but there are lots of healthy liquid alternatives.

Drink up

If you generally start the day with coffee or tea, why not try something more uplifting that will not leave you feeling sluggish by mid-morning? Herbal and fruit teas not only have their own individual tastes but many beneficial health properties too:

Camomile: Long used to help ease digestive problems and calm the nerves. Also said to aid sleep.

Lemon Balm: Relieves tension without causing sleepiness; helps digestion.

Limeflower: Eases stress headaches and also aid sleep.

Rosemary: If you need a pick-me-up for those early mornings, this is the tea to drink as it is known to increase alertness and give energy levels a boost.

Thyme: To lift your spirits, try a cup of thyme.

Morning lift

5fl oz 1 per cent milk

1 teaspoon clear honey

1 banana, chopped

5fl oz natural yogurt

$3^{1}/_{2}$oz frozen berry fruits
(whatever are in season)

Mix all the ingredients together in a blender for a high-protein breakfast drink that will keep your energy levels surging.

Bouncing banana

1 banana, chopped

2 teaspoons lemon juice

1 tablespoon fine oatmeal

2 teaspoons clear honey

3 tablespoons natural yogurt

5fl oz 2 per cent milk

Blend all the ingredients together until smooth.

Lunchtime ideas

Eating a good energy-based lunch can see you through quite happily until your evening meal with no horrendous "lows" on the way. But you must choose energy-based foods. Here are some ideas:

Jacket potato Once regarded as the one of the "bad guys," potatoes have in fact been promoted to the "good guys" list, because it isn't the vegetable that does the damage but rather how it is prepared. A potato is a high-carbohydrate food that contains protein, fiber and vitamin C as well as other essential nutrients, and so it is the ideal lunchtime food. One of the best ways to eat it is in its jacket.

Wash one large potato thoroughly and stab it evenly with a skewer before popping into the microwave (check your microwave instructions for recommended cooking times) or put it into the oven (200°C/400°F) for about 90 minutes.

For some nutritious fillings try:
- 2oz shrimp combined with 2oz sweetcorn, 1 tablespoon salad dressing and 1 tablespoon tomato catsup
- 2oz cooked chicken blended with 1 tablespoon low-fat natural yogurt, diced red and green bell peppers and 1 tablespoon salad dressing
- 4oz tin baked beans with $1/4$ teaspoon chilli powder
- 7oz small tin spaghetti hoops and 2 tomatoes
- Chopped mushrooms fried in a little extra virgin olive oil
- Put 4oz low-fat cottage cheese, 2 tablespoons low-fat yogurt, 1 teaspoon garlic purée and 1 teaspoon dried herbs in a bowl and mix well.

Home-made coleslaw

This recipe makes sufficient for four servings, so store some in the refrigerator for the next day.

1 carrot

3 salad onions

2 red radishes

Stalk of celery

Chunk of crisp lettuce

1 bell pepper (red, green or yellow)

Soy sauce

1 tablespoon cider vinegar

Herb salt (available from healthfood shops)

Black pepper

Wash, peel and grate the vegetables until they are finely shredded. Add in a shake of soy sauce, the cider vinegar, and a sprinkling of salt and pepper. Mix thoroughly. Once the jacket potato is cooked, slice it through the center and pack in a portion of the coleslaw. It's healthy, nutritious, and satisfying!

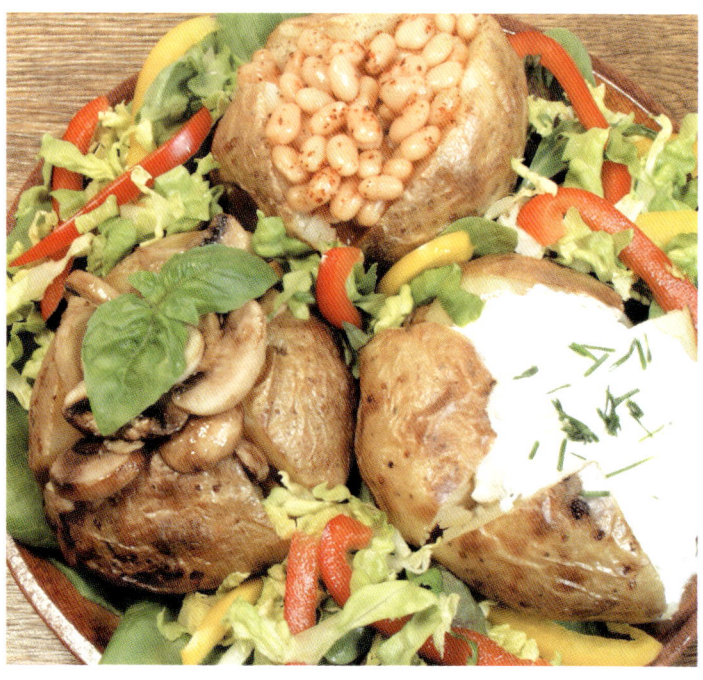

Super sandwiches

Often a sandwich is more appealing at lunchtime than a full meal and can be more convenient, as most cafés, and supermarkets sell them. But although it is easier to buy pre-packaged sandwiches than to make your own, there is always a concern about the ingredients used. So, whenever possible, prepare your own, preferably the night before so there are no excuses the following morning that you haven't time to do it. If they are wrapped in foil, they will keep fresh in the refrigerator overnight.

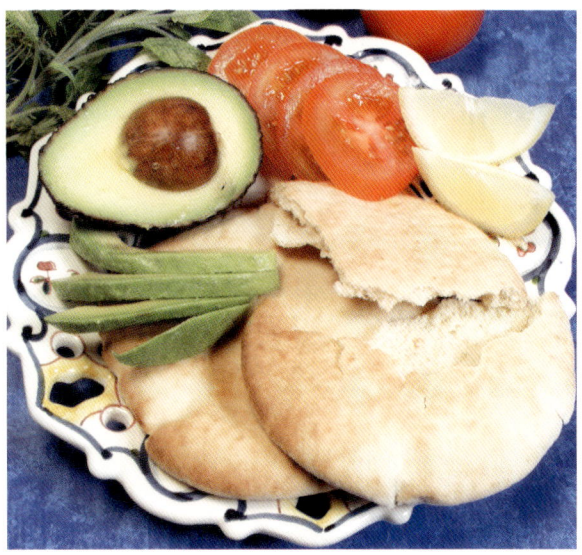

Here are some tasty lunchtime suggestions
- 2 slices of wholemeal bread with tuna and lettuce. Plus an apple
- Pita bread filled with baked beans
- Pita bread with avocado and tomato

Alternatively, try some of these ideas for something a little bit different.

Banana surprise Mash up a banana adding a squeeze of lemon juice. Add crispy bits of bacon and put the mixture between two slices of wholemeal bread.

Fishy treat Drain a tin of sardines or mackerel and mash the fish. Put the mix between two slices of wholemeal bread along with several slices of tomato and some lettuce.

Chicken parcel Perfect if you had chicken for dinner the evening before and still have some cold leftovers. Chop up the chicken and mix it with some low-fat natural yogurt with a few chopped scallions. Place crispy lettuce on two slices of wholemeal bread and spoon the mixture over the top.

Pita celebration Take 1 pita bread, $1/2$ ripe avocado, 1 chopped spring onion, 2 lettuce leaves, 2 tablespoons alfalfa sprouts, 1 sliced tomato, 1 teaspoon vinaigrette dressing, cayenne pepper, and lemon juice. Mash the avocado and scallions in a bowl. Pour in the

vinaigrette dressing and add a pinch of cayenne pepper. When thoroughly blended, spoon the mixture into the pita bread, finishing off with the lettuce leaves, alfalfa sprouts, and tomato. Serve with a squeeze of lemon juice and a pinch of cayenne.

Vegetable surprise

A perfect light lunch on its own or equally as tasty if served to accompany a larger meal.

Small head broccoli
2 carrots
1 leek
1 zucchini
Soy sauce
4oz mozzarella cheese, sliced

Wash the vegetables thoroughly and chop them into small chunks (you can include the broccoli stalks if they are tender). Steam the vegetables until just cooked. Drain well and transfer to a shallow ovenproof dish. Sprinkle over a few drops of soy sauce. Spread the cheese over the top and pop the dish under the broiler until the cheese is golden brown.

Dinnertime recipes

Tasty burgers

8oz cooked chicken, minced
$1/2$ cup onion, grated
$1^1/_2$ cup cottage cheese
1 teaspoon mixed herbs
Salt and black pepper

Mix the chicken and grated onion together in a bowl, then season with salt and pepper. Add the cottage cheese and mixed herbs and stir thoroughly. Shape the mixture into four round burgers and place them on a plate in the refrigerator for 1-2 hours. When you are ready to cook, place the burgers under a hot broiler for approximately 5 minutes for each side. When the burgers are a golden color, serve them with a fresh mixed salad.

Curry in a hurry

This recipe will serve four.
3oz soya chunks (weight when dry)
14oz can tomatoes
1 medium apple, chopped
2 teaspoons pickle
1 teaspoon tomato paste
1 medium onion, chopped
1 bay leaf
1 tablespoon curry powder

Add 2 cups of boiling water to a basin and soak the soya chunks for approximately 10 minutes. Place all the ingredients, together with the soya, in a saucepan and bring to the boil. Cover the saucepan and leave to simmer for 1 hour, occasionally stirring. If the mixture appears slightly thin, remove the lid and increase the heat slightly until the sauce begins to thicken. Serve with brown rice.

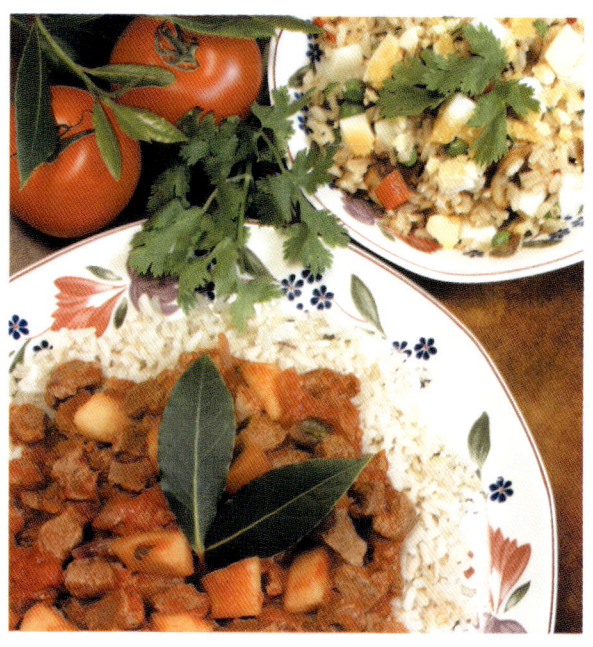

Egg fried rice

1 small onion
1 large mushroom
1 tablespoon virgin olive oil
$1/4$ teaspoon paprika
$1/4$ teaspoon curry powder
1 tablespoon dried herbs
2 large eggs, hard boiled and chopped
Half small red bell pepper
1 cup boiled brown rice
$1/2$ cup cooked petit pois
Soy sauce
Lettuce

Slice the onion and the mushroom and fry in olive oil for 2 minutes. Add the curry powder, paprika, and dried herbs and stir. Shell the eggs and cut into small pieces. Wash and de-seed the red bell pepper and then chop into small pieces. Add the pepper, rice, peas, and soy sauce and heat thoroughly. Before serving, mix in the chopped egg and transfer onto a bed of lettuce.

Delicious desserts

Desserts don't always have to be packed with calories, they can be healthy and great energy boosters. These treats are great for times when you are in a hurry.

Grape salad Scoop out the flesh from half a melon into a dessert dish or tall sundae glass. Take a handful of seedless grapes and cut them in half. Pile them on top of the melon and garnish with sprigs of mint.

Melon shocker Scoop out the flesh from half a melon and put it into a bowl. Add a carton of natural yogurt, stir, and chill before serving.

The whole family will love these delicious desserts. Each recipe serves four.

Mandarin jelly

11 oz can mandarins in natural juice
15fl oz unsweetened orange juice
1 sachet powdered gelatine

Drain the juice from the mandarins and mix with the orange juice. Pour half the liquid into a bowl and sprinkle on the gelatine. Stir well and transfer to a saucepan. Warm gently over a low heat until all the gelatine has dissolved. Add the remaining fruit juice slowly, stirring continuously. Remove from the heat and pour into a bowl. Leave to cool for two minutes before adding the mandarin pieces which will sink to the bottom of the bowl. Cover the bowl and place in the refrigerator until set.

If you feel peckish during the day, eat:
- An orange
- A banana
- Handful of grapes
- Handful of cherries
- Dried fruit
- A carrot
- An apple
- Low-fat yogurt

Pineapple delight

14oz can of crushed pineapple in natural juice
1 packet sugar-free lemon jelly to make 1 pint
5fl oz carton low-fat yogurt

Drain the pineapple and reserve the juice. Follow the instructions to make up the jelly, using the pineapple juice and making the quantity of liquid up to 1 pint. Stir in the crushed pineapple and place in the refrigerator until set. Now for the fun part – once the jelly is firm, use a fork to break it up and then mix in the yogurt. Great on its own or with fresh fruit.

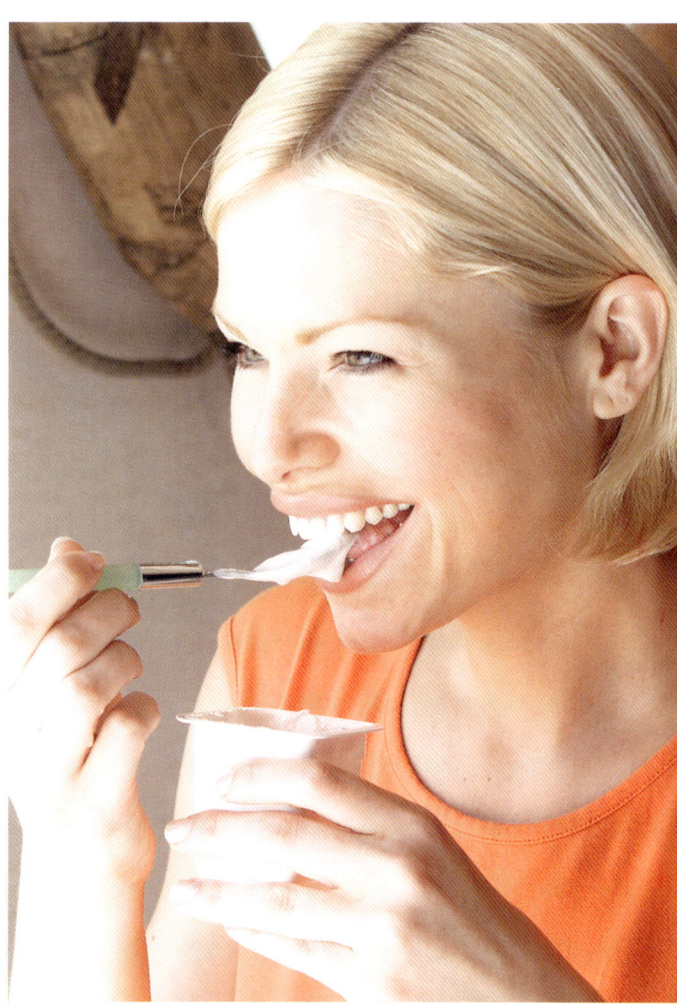

Raise Your Energy

To achieve the ultimate success on the Energize program, which is to feel rejuvenated and invigorated, it is important that you include each of the following elements in your 28-day plan...

Energy shower

There is nothing like an early morning energy shower to kick-start the body into action, so first thing each morning jump into the shower and, if you feel brave enough, when you are about ready to come out, turn the cold faucet full on for a few minutes.

After showering, invigorate your body and boost circulation by slapping yourself all over. Using the flats of your hands and slap from toes to hip, wrist to shoulder and all over your chest, shoulders and torso before rubbing dry with a towel.

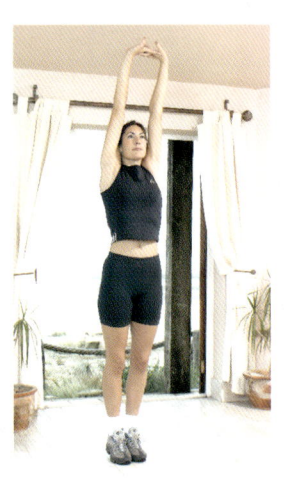

Make sure that each day you:
- Take a daily energy shower
- Do some stretching and flexing of the body at the start of each day
- Spend 30 minutes exercising
- Spend 20 minutes in 'hibernation'
- Spend 5 minutes practicing quality breathing
- Spend 10 minutes hypnotizing yourself
- Each day pamper yourself in some way
- Laugh heartily each day
- Aim to get a good night's sleep

Stretch

A good stretch a day makes aches go away. Try it for yourself. Perform each movement slowly.

1. Link your fingers and raise them above your head until you feel the whole of your upper body stretch.
2. Still keeping your fingers linked, stretch your arms out in front at the same time stretching your back.
3. Place your arms behind you, still with your fingers linked, and as you stretch feel the pull across your chest.
4. Drop your left ear down to your left shoulder, stretching out the muscles of the neck and shoulders, then do the same on the other side.
5. To stretch the back of your neck, drop your chin down to your chest.

Exercise

Exercise to energize. Keep those three words firmly focused in your mind's eye – write them in large print on a piece of paper and pin it up in the kitchen or bathroom so that whenever you feel sluggish, you can remind yourself and keep yourself motivated.

If, apart from walking to the shops, you haven't exercised since the day you left school, then you are bound to feel a little apprehensive. But all the experts advocate a daily dose of physical activity to help us stay emotionally and physically fit. Exercise actually increases energy levels by releasing endorphins which are the body's natural "high" hormones that make you feel great.

Exercising has many other positive benefits:

✓ It gives you greater stamina

✓ It improves posture

✓ It can help you to relax and sleep better

✓ It helps you to deal with everyday stresses more effectively

If you have not exercised for a long while, take it easy at first. Don't overdo it – begin your regime gradually, building up day by day until at the end of the program exercising will have become part of your daily routine.

On the first day or so, just do some gentle exercise, walking to the shops instead of taking the car or getting the bus. Go for a swim or perhaps enroll for a class at your local gym. As your stamina and confidence grow, then you can increase the amount of exercise you take until you actually begin to feel physically tired. The key advice is to participate in activities that you enjoy three times a week, but never to exhaust yourself. If you are stuck for ideas, try some of these:

Jogging, tennis, cycling, skipping. These sports are ideal for raising the heartbeat and should ideally be done for 20 minutes three times a week for a safe energy-building program.

Bouncing. Jogging and jumping on a trampoline is great aerobic exercise. It raises the heartbeat and increases lung capacity without putting unnecessary pressure on knee joints. You could join the local gym or invest in a mini-trampoline to use at home, indoors or out in the garden on days when the weather is good. All the family will be keen to use it!

Walking, swimming, spring-cleaning or digging the garden. These are all forms of exercise that are good for the body. Whatever activity you choose, the most important thing is to do it regularly in order for it to be fully effective. Like most things in life, you only get out what you put in.

Health check

• Before taking up any sport, check with your doctor if you are pregnant or have a medical condition

• Always warm up before starting the routine and cool down slowly after

• Never increase the intensity or length spent exercising if you feel any physical discomfort

• Make sure that you drink plenty of fluids while exercising

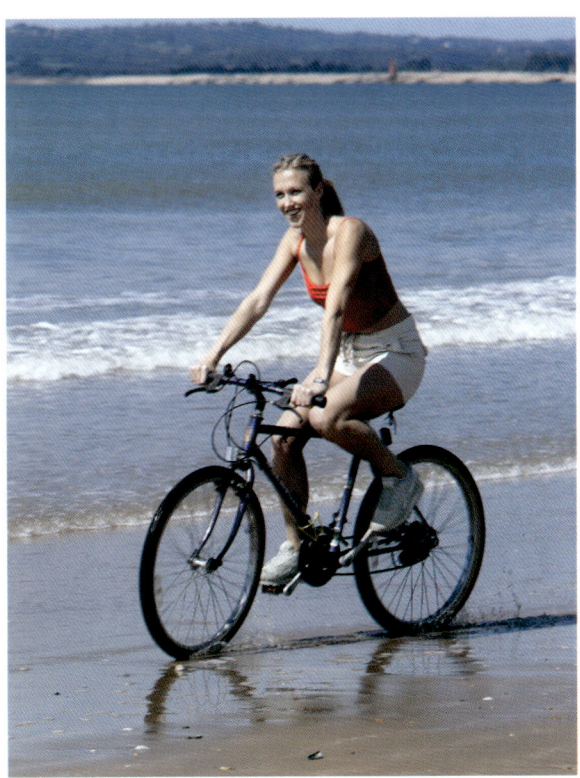

Fact Scientists have discovered that the ideal time of the day to work out is between 4pm and 7pm. According to research, by late afternoon our body temperature, muscle flexibility, and strength have all reached their peak levels.

Restoring Energy

It is amazing how a daily 20-minute mini-break can restore depleted energy resources and recharge flagging batteries.

Hibernation

Simply find a place where you feel totally relaxed and for 20 minutes allow yourself to switch off.

Think about no-one and nothing. Lie down and listen to some favorite music, take a candlelit bath, or even close your eyes and imagine you are a castaway on a desert island with the man of your dreams, and enjoy your 20-minute fantasy!

Deep breathing

There is nothing quite so refreshing or relaxing as five minutes of deep, steady breathing to blow away those cobwebs. And deep breathing is also excellent for helping you to de-stress.

1. Sit in a quiet room.
2. If you are wearing a skirt or pants, undo the waistband so there is ample space for you to expand your stomach.
3. Close your eyes, now slowly breathe in through your nose, holding that breath for a count of five, and then, to a count of five, slowly exhale through your mouth.
4. Repeat this again several times.

Self-hypnotism to combat stress

It is a well-known fact that the growing pressures of everyday modern life have made stress one of the biggest health problems of the age. But on this 28-day program you will learn how to deal with stress; whenever you find yourself in a stressful situation, you will be able to cope if you follow this simple nine-point plan.

1. Make sure that you are alone in the room. Sit down and close your eyes.
2. Say to yourself, "I am going to overcome this tiredness."
3. Now imagine a still river with clear crystal water that tempts you to dive in headfirst.
4. Think of yourself diving into that river and, as you do so, become aware of your tiredness gradually drifting away into the distance like ripples spreading across the surface of the water and getting further and further away.
5. When you can no longer see the ripples, breathe in deeply allowing yourself to float totally free and relaxed.

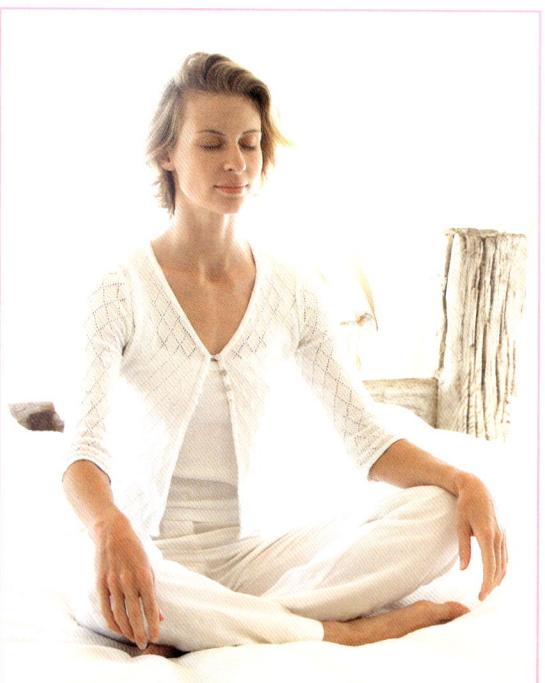

6. Begin stretching your body. Feel every part being stretched gently to its limit, focus your mind's eye on this image.

7. Now imagine that you are sinking deeper and deeper. Allow your body to luxuriate in the sensation of the water as it laps gently around you.

8. Rise up to the surface and bring yourself back to the real world.

9. Breathe out and then breathe in, become conscious of your lungs being filled to their full capacity with air. As you breathe out slowly, be aware that every last bit of stale air is being squeezed out of your lungs. Then open both eyes.

Whenever you feel totally stressed, this is your own secret Shangri-La. It will take several attempts to feel the benefits, but the more your practice, the easier it will become and the more totally relaxed your body will feel.

Laughter

Can you remember the last time you had a jolly good laugh or was it so long ago, you've forgotten? Experts have found that people who use humor to cope with stress experience:
- ✓ Less tension
- ✓ Less fatigue
- ✓ Less anger
- ✓ Less depression

And, furthermore, laughing:
- ✓ Relaxes face muscles
- ✓ Exercises internal muscles
- ✓ Deepens breathing
- ✓ Improves blood circulation
- ✓ Lowers blood pressure and releases endorphins, the feel-good chemicals that are the body's natural painkillers

Or hire a comedy video, read a funny book, or watch your favorite TV sitcom and have a really good laugh.

Sleep

We need sleep almost as much as we need food to fuel our bodies. Without sleep and rest, the body cannot function at its optimum level; it is deprived of the invaluable time it needs to repair cells and recuperate from the rigors of the day. Yet for thousands of people night time is literally a nightmare, a period when they lie awake until the early hours of the morning staring into space. Others spend the entire night tossing and turning in bed and when daylight comes, they are too tired to get up.

Insomnia is a medical condition and there are many drugs and treatments available to help sufferers. However, before going to your doctor, why not try some of these self-help methods?

1. Sleep with the window slightly open.

2. Make sure that the mattress is firm and supportive and that you have sufficient pillows.

3. Eat at least five hours before going to bed.

4. Try and go to bed at the same time every evening.

5. Make sure that you do some exercise during the day. This helps to keep the mind and body active and so ready for rest at night time.

6. Try some relaxation exercises before bedtime.

7. Eat a healthy balanced diet to help your body function more effectively.

Pamper yourself

And why not? You deserve it, you're a good person! Go out and treat yourself to the biggest, brightest bunch of flowers that you can find and if people ask whom they are for, tell them "They're for me, because I deserve them."

Maintaining The Program

There will be times during the 28-day Energize program when you will feel like giving it all up, but such negative thoughts are only to be expected: ignore them. After all, they are only thoughts.

Consider adding some extra treats into your program to provide little rewards to keep yourself motivated. For instance, give yourself a face mask, or how about a foot mask, or pampering yourself with a luxury bath? It's important to keep your spirits up throughout the program. If you get low moments of despondency when you feel exhausted from your daily exercise routine, just remember exercise to energize.

Face mask

Do you ever feel as if your skin could do with some tightening up and that you would love a face mask, but you cannot afford one? Then try this home-made mask which is suitable for all skin types and really does tighten the skin, albeit temporarily.

1. You need one egg and one tablespoon of honey.
2. Separate the egg and beat the white until it is stiff.
3. Add the honey and stir thoroughly.
4. Apply the mixture all over the face and leave it in place for 20 minutes.
5. Rinse it off using warm water.
   If you have particularly dry skin, add several drops of peach kernel oil as a moisturizer.

Foot mask

Your feet are bound to take a lot of punishment once you begin exercising. To keep them in tip-top condition and to prevent the skin from drying out, pamper them with a refreshing foot mask.

1. You need two bananas, two teaspoons of olive oil, two tablespoons of fine sea salt, and the juice of half a lemon.
2. Mash the bananas up in a bowl into which you should then tip the rest of the ingredients.
3. Mix everything thoroughly, rest your feet on a towel, and then massage the mixture into them.
4. Leave it on for approximately ten minutes and then wash it off using warm water.
   Afterwards, apply lots of moisturizer to your feet.

Luxury bath

You will find that there is nothing quite as therapeutic as a luxury bath simply because the essential oils added to the bathwater immediately release calming aromas. Simply add five drops of marjoram and ten drops of lavender oil to a hot bath. Switch off the lights and soak in the bath for a luxurious 20 minutes at least.

Color me happy

Does wearing a bright red T-shirt make you feel happy or sad? Or do you feel calm when wearing a green sweater? According to scientists, colors can have a strong effect upon our emotions, and so bringing color into one's life can really help to lift the spirits and alleviate feelings of lethargy.

When energy levels are low, you inevitably feel a little downhearted and nothing seems to feel or look right on you. So when, halfway through the program, you find you begin to feel in need of cheering up, treat yourself to a new T-shirt, some pretty flowers, or even a new lamp to brighten up your living room or bedroom!

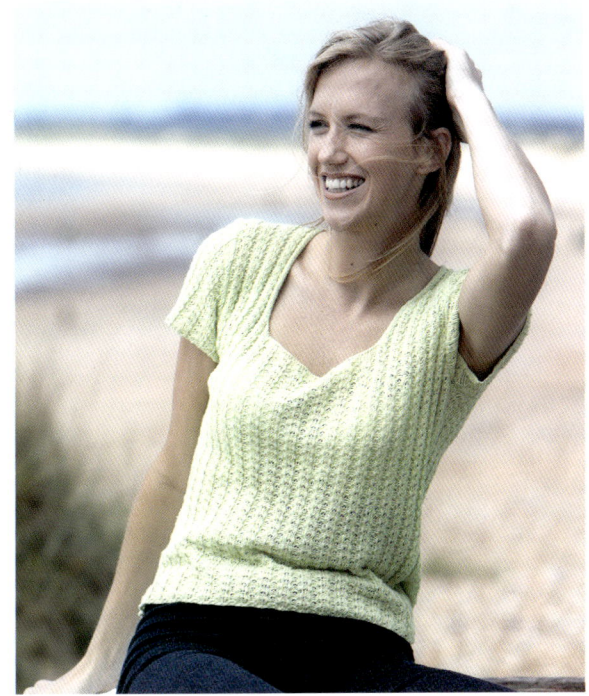

Certain colors can influence your feelings:
Blue: Invokes a feeling of calm.
Green: A soothing color, one that is said to alleviate feelings of anxiety or fear.
Orange: Enhances enthusiasm, creativity, and courage.
Red: Gives of a sense of warmth and excitement.
Violet: Improves self-confidence and encourages intuitive thinking.
Yellow: Promotes hope, happiness, and consideration.

Think positive

You may well face days during the program when you feel down, but hidden beneath those feelings are positive emotions lying in wait. Every day, try to work hard to bring them to the surface. When you feel good about yourself, you can begin to understand the type of person you are and accept your characteristics, even your imperfections. Experts have found that people who are positive and optimistic usually enjoy long-term good health.

How to lift negative emotions
• Keep a diary of those negative thoughts, write them down at the end of the day and then start to challenge them by putting positive messages alongside. "I don't feel that I am any more energetic" might be the negative message, "but you are doing a lot more than before" could be a positive reply.
• If you have times when you feel anxious or stressed out, stop and think about happy occasions and try to remember how they felt.
• Ignore negative thoughts whenever they worm their way into your mind. After all, millions of thoughts pass through our minds each day; thoughts can't harm you.
• Why not set yourself a challenge while on the program – take up a new sport and aspire to a certain level of proficiency. By achieving this, you will feel much more confident of your abilities.

Energize: Days 1–7

You've done all the preparatory work and now can look forward to the 28-day Energize program. By the end it you should feel invigorated and rejuvenated. Whether you are a working woman or a busy mother at home, the next 28 days should witness some of the biggest changes that you will ever make to your life...so be prepared!

Draw up a chart (see page 31) and stick it on your fridge or kitchen wall so that you will remember exactly what you must include on each day of your 28 day program.

Keep a diary and record in it all the day's activities, what you ate, how you felt when you woke up, how you relaxed. At the end of each day summarize how you feel. Naturally on some days you will find more to write about than on others, but it will help to keep you motivated if you keep this diary and refer to it for encouragement when you have down days. Weigh yourself today only!

Here is a typical plan for day 1, but of course times and the order in which activities are done may differ, according to your individual lifestyle and work commitments.

6.45am Aim to get up 20 minutes earlier than normal. Kick-start the body by drinking a glass of hot water with a squeeze of lemon added to it.
7.15am Spend ten minutes stretching and flexing the whole body.
8.00am Take an energy shower or bath, slapping the skin before towelling yourself dry.
8.45am Time for breakfast. Have some wheatgerm with yogurt, honey, and stewed dried apricots and a cup of lemon herbal tea. Eat the meal slowly so that you can savor each mouthful.
9.30am Go for a brisk 30-minute walk.
11.00am Have a glass of water and then do some deep breathing.
1.00pm Lunch – a jacket potato filled with spaghetti hoops and two tomatoes. Finish with an apple.
2.15pm Practice some self-hypnosis. Have a glass of herbal tea.
4.00pm Time for some pampering – treat your feet to a foot mask.
6.00pm Prepare the evening meal. Perhaps try a vegetable curry tonight.
7.00pm Time for hibernation.
8.00pm Have a pleasant luxury bath and then get ready for an early night.

Don't forget: As you complete each activity, tick it off on your chart and before you go to sleep remember to record in your diary how you felt, noting down both the good and the bad points.

Remainder of the week

The remainder of the first week should more or less follow the pattern established here, but remember to add different foods and try some different exercises. If you feel a little bored by day 6, do something totally out of character – you're allowed to! How about buying yourself a huge colored ball and persuading a family member or friend to have a game of "Pass The Ball" in the garden, or see how many times you can bounce it in the air. Not only are you getting exercise, but you're having fun too. Sometimes mad moments like this are great for de-stressing the mind and body.

Exercise diary

It is a good idea to keep an exercise diary. Make a note of the activities you have undertaken and how you felt afterwards and you will soon begin to see clear signs of improvement in stamina and fitness. Fill it in at the end of each day and by the end of the program you will see how much more you are able to do than at the beginning.

Energy snacks

While on the 28-day energy program, you may well find yourself feeling peckish from time to time, or experiencing withdrawal symptoms from the lack of sugar in your diet. In this case it is always a good idea to have some nibbles on hand which can help stave off those hunger pangs and raise energy levels.

All the following are good energy snacks:

- Bananas
- Dried fruit
- Fresh fruit
- Nuts – brazil, flaked almonds, pecans, pine, walnuts
- Raw vegetables
- Oatcakes
- Pumpkin seeds
- Rice cakes
- Sunflower seeds

Instant energizers

When you are stressed, your breathing will almost inevitably quicken. It becomes shallow and in doing so prevents the lungs from taking in a full quota of oxygen. This ultimately leads to tiredness. To remedy this there are several instant remedies:
- Sit still for several minutes, breathing in through the nose slowly for a count of four and then out through the mouth for a count of four.
- Shake your hands vigorously from side to side.
- With the forefinger and thumb, massage around the rims of both ear lobes.

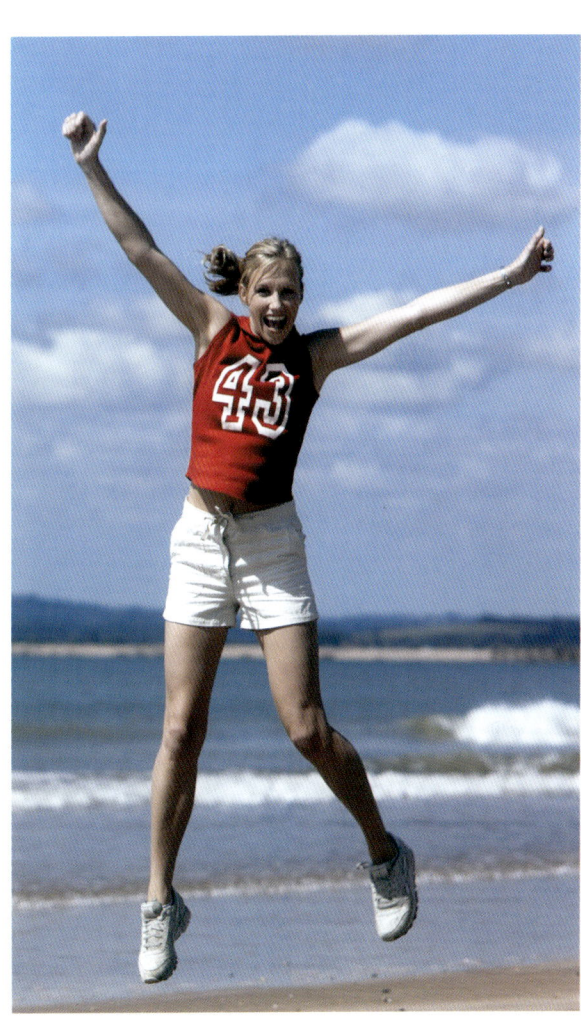

Energize: Days 8–14

By now you will have established a routine and perhaps made some changes to personalize the program to suit your lifestyle. So are you ready for week two?

6.45am Kick-start the body with a glass of hot water and add a squeeze of lime juice.

7.15am Spend 10 minutes stretching and flexing.

8.00am Take an energy shower or bath, slapping the skin before towelling yourself dry.

8.45am Time for breakfast. Mix a chopped banana and a small pot of low-fat yogurt with some unsweetened muesli.

9.30am Buy yourself a skipping rope and spend 20 minutes skipping – remember to warm up gradually. Do not skip on a very hard surface as it may put strain on joints and muscles.

11.00am Have a glass of water and take time to do some quality breathing.

1.00pm Lunch. A chicken salad might be nice.

2.15pm Why not hire a comedy video or treat yourself to an afternoon at the cinema if there is a comedy showing. It's good to laugh. Take some dried fruit for snacking.

4.00pm Have a glass of fresh juice and do an instant energizer (see page 27).

6.00pm Evening meal. Maybe burgers tonight.

7.00pm Give your hair a home-made conditioning treatment.

8.00pm Hibernate for 20 minutes before getting an early night with a good book.

Don't forget: As you complete each activity, tick it off on your chart. Before you go to sleep, remember to record in your diary how you felt, writing down both the good and the bad points.

Remainder of the week

The remainder of week 2 should follow the same basic routine more or less. Once again, vary what you eat and your schedule for the following day – adding subtle changes will help to ensure that you don't get bored.

Avocado hair conditioner
This recipe is suitable for all hair types.
- Take one avocado.
- Remove the stone from the avocado and mash the flesh into a soft pulp.
- Massage the mixture into the hair and scalp.
- Cover the hair with a plastic bag and leave it for a full hour.
- Shampoo and rinse as normal.

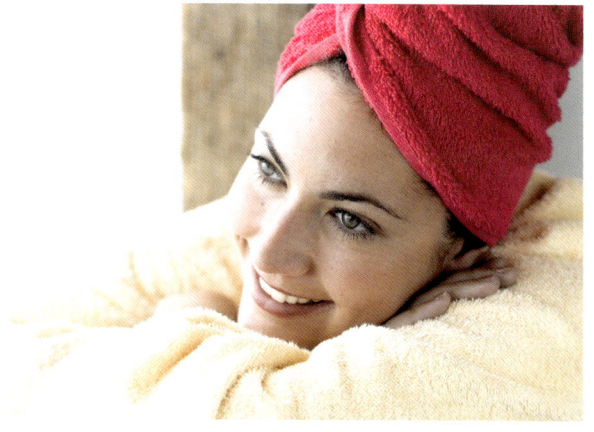

Energize: Days 15–21

You are halfway there! Take a moment to congratulate yourself and then get ready for week three. You have probably established quite a fixed routine by now – remember to add changes and variations to the daily schedule to keep things fresh.

6.45am Kick-start the body with a glass of hot water and add a squeeze of lemon juice.

7.15am Spend 10 minutes stretching and flexing.

8.00am Take an energy shower or bath, slapping the skin before towelling yourself dry.

8.45am Time for breakfast. Start today with a muffin topped with fat-free cheese and a glass of freshly squeezed orange juice.

9.30am Do some gardening, or pop along to the shops, making sure you walk there and back briskly.

11.00am Have a glass of herbal tea and spend 20 minutes meditating.

1.00pm Try a new lunch dish today.

2.15pm Practice a session of self-hypnotism. Afterwards, sit down, relax and read a book or listen to some music.

4.00pm Have a glass of fresh juice and do an instant energizer.

6.00pm Evening meal. Egg fried rice is good.

7.00pm If you've had a busy day, your eyes may be feeling tired, so treat them to some pampering (see the eye revival recipe).

8.00pm Spend time quality breathing. If you are feeling peckish, eat a piece of fruit and watch some TV before going to bed.

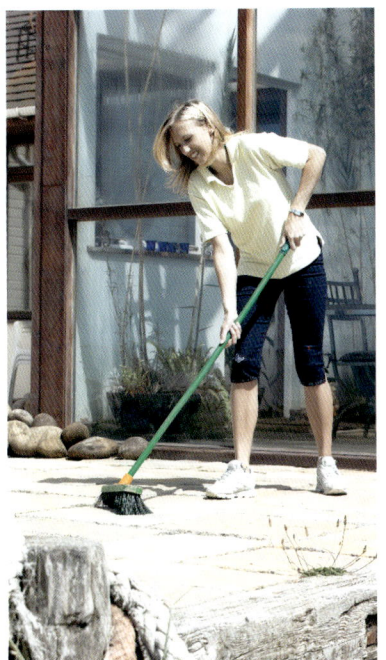

Don't forget: As you complete each activity, tick it off on your chart. Before you go to sleep, remember to record in your diary how you felt, writing down both the good and the bad points.

Remainder of the week

Keep up with the routine even if on some days you don't feel like it. If you really feel down in the dumps, do something positive to break the mood. Go along to your local gym for a workout, and don't forget that a good dose of brisk housework or gardening is just as beneficial as a 35-minute swim in the pool.

Eye revival recipe
For puffy tired eyes.
- Take a quarter of a cucumber and one teaspoon of powdered milk.
- Grate enough cucumber, to measure approximately two teaspoons in quantity.
- Add one teaspoon of powdered milk.
- Mix together so it forms a paste. Apply it to both eyelids and also along the lower part of the eye socket.
- Leave it for ten minutes before sponging off with damp absorbent cotton.

Energize: Days 22–28

This is it! You are nearing the end of your 28-day Energize program and you have survived. You should begin to feel more energetic now, largely on account of a healthier diet combined with regular exercise and relaxation. So don't give up now. Why throw away all your hard-won gains?

6.45am Kick-start the body with a glass of hot water and add a squeeze of lemon juice.

7.15am Spend 10 minutes stretching and flexing the body.

8.00am Take an energy shower or bath, slapping the skin before towelling yourself dry.

8.45am Time for breakfast. Scrambled egg on rye bread.

9.30am Go for a brisk walk and work up a sweat.

11.00am Have a glass of herbal tea and spend five minutes concentrating on quality breathing.

1.00pm Lunch – pita bread and beans is delicious.

2.15pm Go into town and buy yourself a brightly colored vest or perhaps a bright new plant as a reward. Make sure that it is bright and cheerful. Sit down and have a glass of water when you get home. If you are feeling peckish, have some nuts.

4.00pm Time for 20 minutes hibernation.

6.00pm Evening meal. You might decide to go out for dinner to celebrate your success. Remember to choose healthily. After dinner go to the pictures and, if it's not a comedy, then perhaps see a weepy. Often a good cry is as relaxing as a good laugh.

10.00pm Bed and the sleep of the just!

Don't forget: As you complete each activity, tick it off on your chart. Before you go to sleep, remember to record in your diary how you felt, writing down both the good and the bad points.

Remainder of the week

Keep up with the routine right through to the very last day. On the final day why not celebrate, and treat yourself to some new exercise clothes? If you are feeling really good, from now on exercise will become part of your daily life.

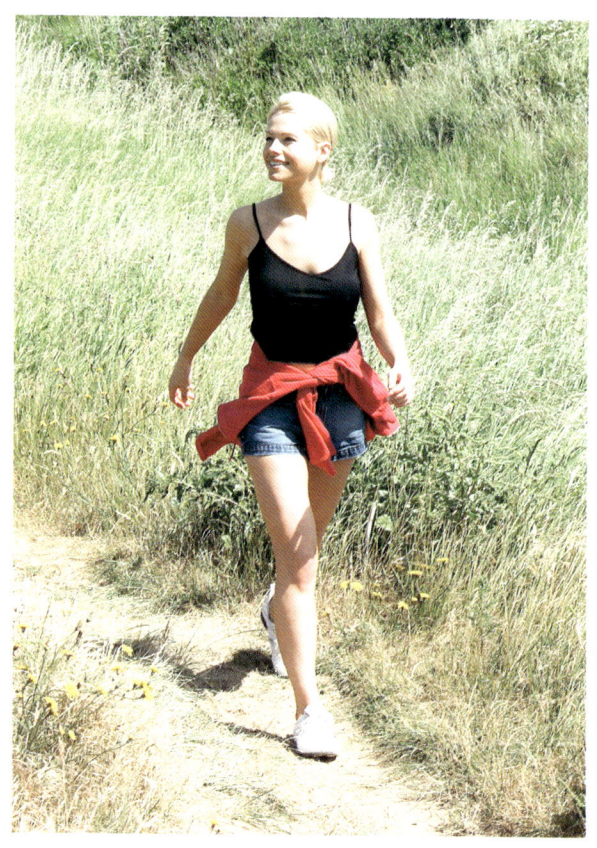

Activity Record Chart

Record your activities every day using this table

DAILY ACTIVITIES	1	2	3	4	5	6	7	8	9	10	11	12	13	14	15	16	17	18	19	20	21	22	23	24	25	26	27	28
Glass of hot water and lemon or lime juice																												
Stretch and flex																												
Energy shower																												
Breakfast																												
Lunch																												
Dinner																												
One dose of aloe vera																												
3 pints water																												
Multivitamin supplement																												
3 portions of fresh fruit																												
3 servings of vegetables																												
1 portion non-dairy product																												
20 mins hibernation																												
10 mins self-hypnotism																												
30 mins exercise																												
Pampering																												
5 mins breathing																												
Laugh																												

Congratulations!

You've done it! You've successfully completed the 28-day Energize program. You will probably feel healthier now than you have done for ages and very proud of yourself too.

Not only have you succeeded in eating more healthily, but you have also learned how to energize your body by exercising. You'll now know much more about your own body than you ever thought possible.

There have almost certainly been moments in the last 28 days when you felt unable to go on, but you didn't let those moments of self-doubt stand in your way and you should be very proud of yourself. And now that you have achieved this peak of good health, make sure you hold on to it.

After all, you are the only person who can make sure that you do!

To keep energy levels high:
- Avoid refined foods, such as white rice, sugar, and bread
- Cut out stimulants, such as coffee, chocolate, or sugar
- Eat regular small meals and healthy snacks throughout the day
- Increase your intake of complex carbohydrates – brown rice, wholegrains, and seeds – which release energy slowly and steadily
- Include a protein food, such as chicken, fish or, for vegetarians, quorn or tofu with each meal
- Don't skip breakfast

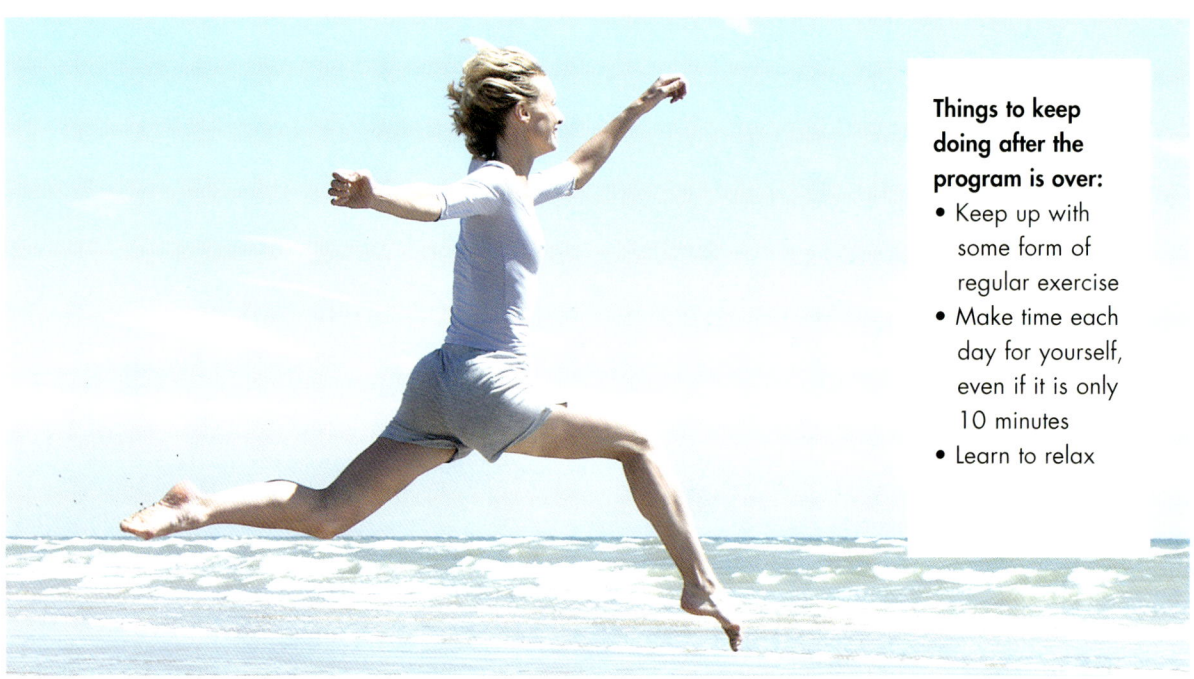

Things to keep doing after the program is over:
- Keep up with some form of regular exercise
- Make time each day for yourself, even if it is only 10 minutes
- Learn to relax